Sex! What's That?

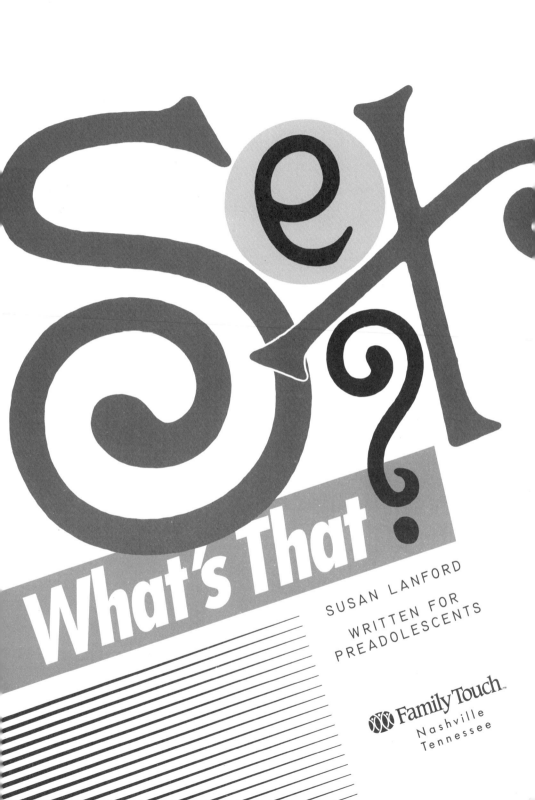

Sex: What's That?

SUSAN LANFORD

WRITTEN FOR PREADOLESCENTS

Family Touch™

Nashville
Tennessee

7807-43
ISBN: 0-8054-9967-9

Dewey Decimal Classification: 155.3
Subject Heading: SEX EDUCATION//SEXUAL BEHAVIOR
Printed in the United States of America

Family Touch Press
127 Ninth Avenue, North
Nashville, TN 37234

Contents

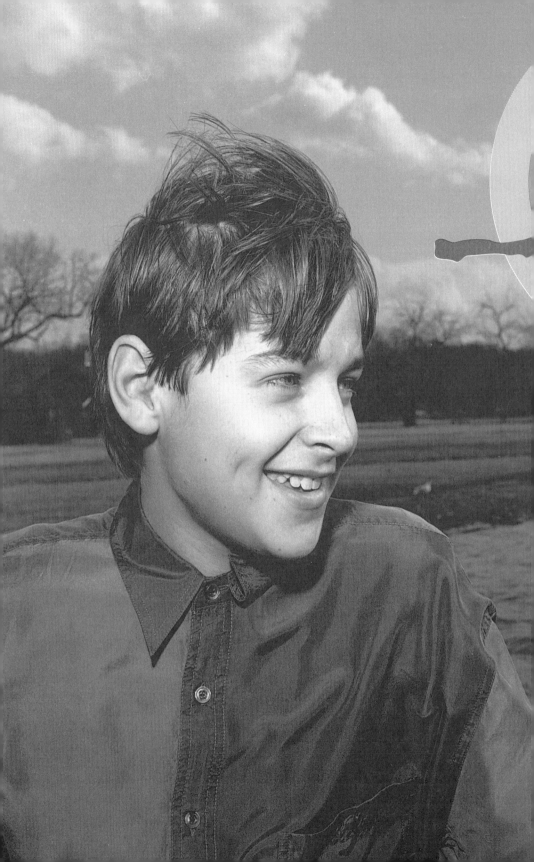

Preadolescent— and Proud of It

Welcome to the wonderful world of preadolescence! Don't worry about that big word—*preadolescent*. It's not a disease.

You're a smart guy or gal, I'm guessing. Suppose *you* figure this puzzle out:

pre: coming before

adolescence: the teenage years, usually beginning at age *twelve*

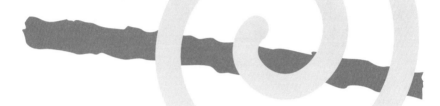

That makes *you* a...well, let's see, that means you're a...a *teenager under construction*. That's it! I mean, that's you!

Perhaps you've heard adults talk about being "between jobs." As a preadolescent, you're "between stages" in your growth. You're between childhood and your teenage years.

Now, if you looked yourself up in a college textbook, it would label your age as "late childhood" or "early adolescence." Your church may call your group "older children" or "younger youth." At school, some of you are "older elementary school kids," "middle schoolers," or "junior highers." There may be times you grump around the house because it seems your parent is treating you like a little kid and you feel older than that.

These *books* and *people* and *you* know that you are no longer any ordinary kid. There are changes beginning in your body and in your feelings. You're making tougher choices about what to do and with whom to do it. You're really between childhood and adolescence.

So, isn't it great that these years have a special name—preadolescence? I hope that helps you know that you're special at this age, just as you are at every age.

Even though you are in a "between" stage, don't think that it is some no man's land. Your stage already has a nickname—"the tweens." It makes sense, and it's easier to say than preadolescence.

There are music groups that play just for the tween crowd. Special clothing lines are made for preteens. Parents' magazines have special sections on understanding tweens.

Preadolescent, preteen, tween... they all mean the same person— YOU. And this book is just for you.

As you read, you may see some words and not be sure about their meaning. Some of these words will be explained where they are first used. If you find one that is not explained, ask your parents or an adult friend.

I also want you to know that we are fortunate. The Bible has a lot to say about being created by God, being male or female, taking care of your body, and acting in ways that please God. I'll be sharing many Bible passages with you. When I do, there will be a headline that includes this phrase:

THINK ON THESE THINGS

I took that phrase from one of my favorite Bible verses. It says:

"Whatever is true, whatever is noble, whatever is right, whatever is pure, whatever is lovely, whatever is admirable—if anything is excellent or praiseworthy—think about such things" (Phil.4:8, NIV).

(The *King James Version* of the Bible says "think on these things.")

That's the way I want you to learn about yourself and your sexuality—by thinking on these things from God's point of view. I don't know of a better way.

Also, I have included space in the back of this book for you to write down new ideas you discover in each chapter and list questions that you still need answered. I encourage you to use this section, "My Journal—Ideas and Questions," beginning on page 74 as a way to follow-up our discussion. Then, talk with a parent or trusted adult friend about any concerns or questions that remain.

As I write, I think constantly about my thirteen-year-old son, and my eleven-year-old daughter, both *super* kids I might add. I'm writing just as if they and I were talking. As you read, imagine we're talking together too—you and I. Ready? Let's talk!

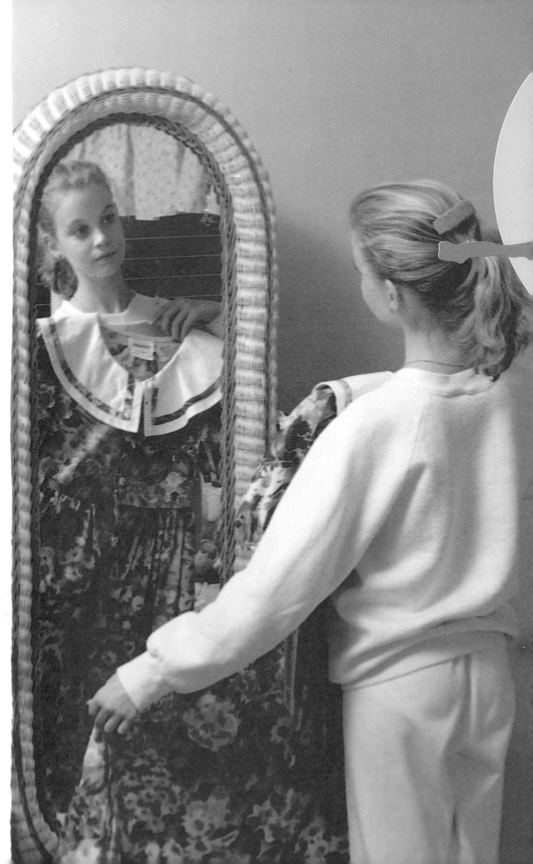

My Body—What It Means to Be Me

We *could* talk about sex right off the bat! How embarrassing, you may be thinking. OK, we won't talk about sex yet. That's a word that means many different things to different people. And it's one of those "red-flag" words—hard to discuss sometimes.

Here's where we really need to start talking. Let's talk about *sexuality*.

Sexuality is another formal-sounding word (like preadolescence—remember?). When we talk about your sexuality, we're talking about…

… what makes you different from others

… what it means to be a boy or a girl

… what it means to be *you*.

God best understands all this. Remember, you were His idea!

SEXUALITY… THINK ON THESE THINGS

◆ It's as old as creation.

> "When God created man, he made him in the likeness of God. He created them male and female and blessed them" (Gen. 5:1-2, NIV).

From the beginning, God meant for there to be two types of people, **male** and **female**. This is part of God's original design for how the world should be. People—men and women, boys and girls—are our constant reminders that God is creative.

◆ We're the *best* of creation.

Read the story of creation in Genesis 1. At several points in describing God's creation, the Bible says,

> "And God saw that it [what He had created] was good" (Gen. 1:10,12,18,21, 25, NIV).

At the end of the sixth day, when man and woman were created, the Bible says,

> "God saw all that He had made, and it was very good" (Gen. 1: 31, NIV).

Only people are made in God's image. Only people are capable of knowing and loving God, and being known and loved by Him. Long ago, David exclaimed:

> "You made him [meaning "people"] a little lower than the heavenly beings and crowned him with glory and honor.
> "You made him ruler over the works of your hands;
> you put everything under his feet:
> all flocks and herds, and the beasts of the field, the birds of the air, and the fish of the sea...,
> "O Lord, our Lord, how majestic is your name in all the earth!" (Ps. 8:5-9, NIV).

◆ Marriage and sex—two gifts in the *same* package.

Genesis 2 tells about Adam and Eve. Jesus quoted Genesis 2:24 to teach about marriage. Because people are created male and female, Jesus said people marry and "become one flesh" (Gen. 2:24; Matt. 19:5, NIV). "Become one flesh" is a biblical phrase. Today, you might hear the phrases "have sex," "make love," or "sexual intercourse." All refer to the physical union of a man and a woman. But the Bible phrase "become one flesh" means more than just a physical union.

It means that a husband and wife...
... care deeply for each other
... share every part of their lives with each other
... believe that their marriage is a gift from God
... express all these feelings and beliefs through physical touch, closeness, and the act of sexual intercourse.

Between husbands and wives, sex is a gift from God. It is a good, delightful gift. Remember the verse about Adam and Eve:

"The man and his wife were both naked, and they felt no shame" (Gen. 2:25, NIV).

They knew that their bodies, including their sexual parts, were created by God. And they knew they were created for each other.

You can look forward to that gift. God's gift of marriage includes God's gift of sex with your husband or your wife.

My Tween Body...What's Going On?

Matthew thinks his gang of twelve-year-old friends is falling apart. Everyone is getting too weird! Zac has a few fuzzy hairs on his upper lip and thinks he's the greatest. Phil has turned into such a grouch since his face broke out. Jonathan is absolutely loopy over Jessica. And whenever Matthew wants to ride bikes with Michael, he's either eating or sleeping.

Kristin is confused, too. She and her two best friends are taller than the boys in class. Casy is fighting with her mom over everything. Rachel is the only 10-year-old at school wearing a bra, and she thinks she's better than everyone else. And whenever Jonathan talks to Jessica, she drops her books, trips on her shoelaces, or does something else just as klutzy.

What's going on?

The *good news* is this:

The physical changes in all these kids are *normal*. Just like what's happening to you is normal. YOU ARE A NORMAL PERSON.

The *better news* is this:

These are the healthiest years of your life. You've probably already survived those kid diseases, like measles and chicken pox. Your body has made extra protection to fight infections. In fact, you now have twice as much of this protection as any adult. No wonder you hate wearing heavy coats and love playing in the rain.

The *best news* is this:

Even though you and your body are changing, some things will never change. You are still the basic *you*. Your parents still love you. God loves and understands you. And that's the *very best* news of all.

YOU ARE CHANGING, BUT FIRST...

THINK ON THESE THINGS

▼ God created you, the individual, one-of-a-kind you. David praised Him for this by saying:

"For you created my inmost being; you knit me together in my mother's womb.

"...all the days ordained for me were written in your book before one of them came to be" (Ps. 139:13,16, NIV).

▼ God deliberately designed and made your body, including the sexual parts. Paul said:

"God has arranged the parts in the body, every one of them, just as he wanted them to be" (1 Cor. 12:18, NIV).

▼ Your body, changing and growing, may be a mystery to you, but it's not a mystery to God. David learned this and said:

"O Lord, you have searched me and you know me.

"I praise You because I am fearfully and wonderfully made;
your works are wonderful, I know that full well" (Ps. 139:1,14, NIV).

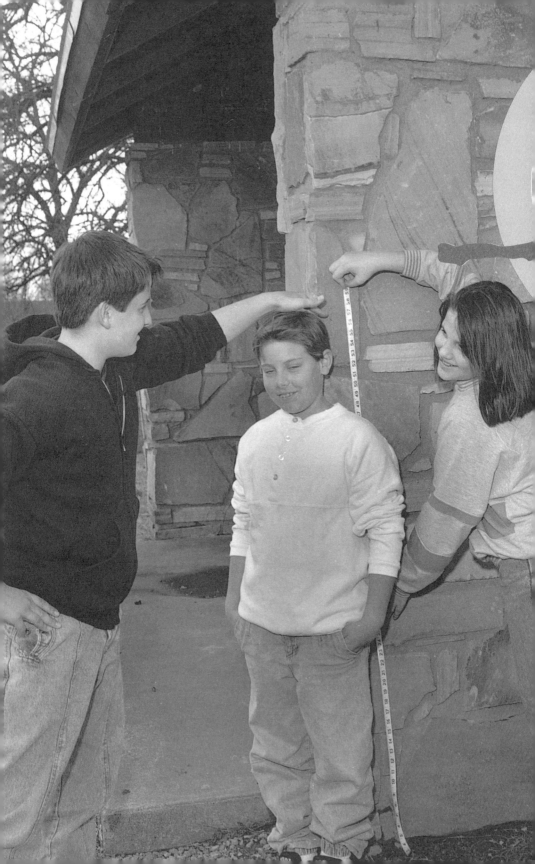

My Growing— Understanding God's Timing

In the grocery store nowadays, you can buy a roasting hen or turkey with a pop-up timer. The cooking instructions help you guess how much time the bird will need to cook. But the proof of doneness for the cook is that timer. When it pops, it's time to stop cooking and start eating.

God created you with something like a pop-up timer.

It is your *pituitary gland*, a tiny organ at the base of your brain. This timer is set to pop at a different time for you than for your friends. The timing of this gland's work explains all the physical and emotional differences in Matthew and Kristin and their friends.

The pituitary gland releases chemical messages, called *hormones*, into your body.

One hormone controls the growth of your body.

These are the sorts of body changes you can expect right now:
★ growing taller
★ getting heavier
★ hands and feet growing before the rest of your body grows
★ bones growing faster than muscles (that's why you are surprised at how clumsy you are sometimes)
★ pimples appearing
★ beginnings of body odor, especially after physical exercise or play

These changes could start anytime between ages nine to fourteen. Most girls will start these changes two years before most boys. Some days you may wish your growth would hurry up or slow down. Remember, your body is following God's plan for it. Your worry won't change the way you grow.

Now, *another* hormone controls changes in your sexuality. You will also notice changes like:

For girls
- a rounder, softer body
- breasts beginning to round, and the nipples starting to darken
- hair growing in the pubic area and under the arms
- menstruation, a monthly flow of blood from the uterus and vagina, begins

For boys
- a more solid, bonier body
- testicles growing larger as they begin to make sperm cells
- the penis becoming bigger
- hair growing around the penis and on the upper lip
- the penis sometimes becoming hard and stiff; this is called an erection

You may not know what some of these terms mean. Let's define the sexual organs and learn what they do.

For girls

Uterus—This pear-shaped organ inside the lower abdomen is about three inches across. It is the place babies grow for nine months. The uterus stretches as the baby gets bigger, and then shrinks to its original size after the baby is born.

Fallopian Tubes—There are two, one on each side of the uterus. A mature egg cell travels through one of these tubes to the uterus each month. When an egg cell is joined by a sperm cell, we say the egg is fertilized. This joining of an egg cell and a sperm cell usually will happen in one of the fallopian tubes.

Ovaries—The ovaries are two almond-shaped glands at the end of each fallopian tube. Ovaries produce and store thousands of egg cells. An egg cell is also called an ovum.

Ovaries also produce hormones which help a girl's body change to a woman's body. These hormones also prepare her uterus each month for the egg cell which travels to it.

Vagina—This is the passageway from the uterus to the outside of the body. The walls of the vagina also stretch and shrink, since a baby travels from the uterus through the vagina to be born. After puberty, the monthly flow of blood (menstruation) also travels through the vagina to the outside of the body.

Vulva—These are folds of skin between a girl's legs which cover the vagina. The **urethra**, where urine is passed out of the body, is also inside the vulva.

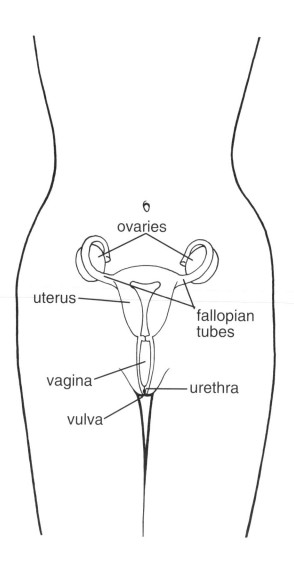

ovaries

uterus — fallopian tubes

vagina — urethra

vulva

Girls, it is important to keep the vulva and the opening of your vagina clean. Once your sex glands begin releasing hormones into your body, you may notice a new odor at times from this area of your body. A gentle, daily washing as you bathe or shower will be important. This is especially true during menstruation. Do not try to clean inside your vagina or try to poke anything into it. Just carefully wash the folds of skin of the vulva and the opening of the vagina. And, after a bowel movement, carefully wipe yourself from front to back, away from your urethra and vagina. Otherwise, bacteria may start an infection that will make you sick.

For boys

Testicles—You have two of them. They are glands. In them, sperm cells are made. The testicles of a grown man will produce billions of sperm in a month's time. The testicles also produce hormones which change a boy's body into the body of a man.

Scrotum—This is a bag of skin. The testicles are inside it, separated from each other by a thin membrane. The scrotum hangs between the legs and behind the penis.

Sperm Ducts—Sperm are stored in these tubes which run from each testicle to the penis. There are two sperm ducts.

Seminal Vessel and **Prostate Gland**—These two small glands help the male body make semen. This is the milky-white liquid which

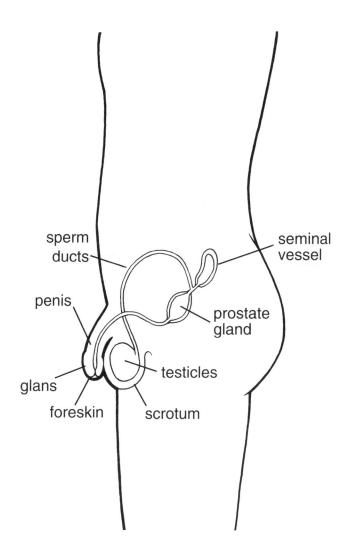

sperm ducts

seminal vessel

penis

prostate gland

glans

testicles

foreskin

scrotum

carries sperm through the penis and out of the body.

Penis—The soft, fleshy organ between the legs. It passes urine which travels to it through the urethra, a small tube leading from the bladder.

For semen to pass through the penis, it must be erect. The tissue of the penis has many empty spaces. When blood fills these spaces, the penis stands out from the body; it is longer and firm. This is an erection. The passing of semen is called ejaculation. Urine does not pass through the penis during ejaculation. You've already read about these two things.

The penis needs to be washed and kept clean, especially the tip, called the **glans**. Otherwise, the glans may itch or become sore. The glans is covered by an extra piece of skin called **foreskin**. Some boys have an operation at birth called circumcision; the doctor cut off the foreskin. Whether you are circumcised or uncircumcised, you are a normal boy. Boys who were not circumcised should carefully pull back the foreskin to bathe the glans.

Whew again! That's a lot of information. But isn't it remarkable how complex God created our bodies? And isn't it wonderful how everything necessary for life to begin and grow is given to us? God trusts us with *life itself*. King David marveled at God's knowledge of everything about him. He wrote,

"Such knowledge is too wonderful for me, too lofty for me to attain" (Ps. 139:6, NIV).

Now, check yourself to see how much you remember. Point to each word in the list. Try to recall:

◆ Whether the body part is a *male* or a *female* part.
◆ *How many* are in one person's body.

If you are not sure of your answers, check back through this chapter.

❑ fallopian tube ❑ foreskin

❑ glans ❑ ovary

❑ testicles ❑ penis

❑ prostate gland ❑ scrotum

❑ urethra ❑ seminal vessel

❑ sperm duct ❑ uterus

❑ vagina ❑ vulva

OK, I hear you gasping in the background. Maybe a little too much too fast through here? You might try getting used to that feeling, because you will have days when it seems everything about you—your body, your feelings, your friends—is growing and changing.

We're still talking about the kind of growing you can expect, sometime between ages nine and fourteen. I'd like to talk about the one change which is most noticeable to you preadolescents. For girls, it is your period, or menstruation. For boys, it is a wet dream, or nocturnal emission.

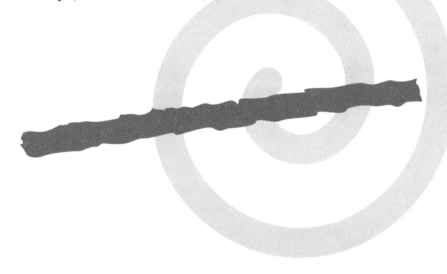

Girls, the major physical change that tells you your body is changing to a woman's body is *menstruation*. Let me ask some questions you may be thinking and give you some answers.

Q **"How does it happen?"**

A Good idea! Let's start with the basics. Your body produces a special cell, called an *egg cell*, in your ovaries. This egg cell could begin a new life, a baby, if it joins with a sperm cell which males produce. Girls, when an egg cell travels toward your uterus, the uterus prepares for its arrival by producing a soft inside lining and extra blood. This would nourish a new baby. But when no sperm cell joins the egg cell, a baby does not grow, and the extra lining in your uterus is not needed.

Then, the egg cell and the extra lining and blood in your uterus leave your body through your vagina. This flow will look like blood—most of it is blood. It takes three to seven days for this flow to finish.

Your parents or teachers may call this "getting your period" or "starting your period." Your periods may be unpredictable for a while and not stick to a schedule. It will probably start at times or in places you wish it wouldn't. I know that can be embarrassing.

After a few months, usually no more than a year, you may be able to predict when your period will start. In fact, you may want to keep track of it on a calendar in your room. Generally, there are twenty-eight to thirty days between the start of one period and the start of the next.

Q **"I want to be ready for this first period. How do I know it's coming?"**

A Good question. Menstruation generally starts about two years after your breasts begin to grow. This is a very gradual change, and you won't be able to pin down an exact starting date. Watch for all the other body changes I mentioned earlier—rounder, softer body, hair growing in the pubic area and under your arms. These are all signs your body is changing from a girl's to a woman's, and your period will begin after these changes take place.

Q **"When I cut myself, blood means I'm hurt and I try to stop it. Is this the same?"**

A Another good question. The blood of your period means it was not needed inside your uterus to nourish a growing baby. Its flow outside of you means you're a normal girl, not that you're hurt. You won't want to stop it; you'll want to catch it. You will use a *sanitary napkin*, a cotton pad worn inside your panties, or a *tampon* a small cotton roll placed inside your vagina. Your mom or another woman friend can help you choose what you will use and help you know how often to change it.

Q **"Every month!—for how long?"**

A Menstruation stops in mid-life, probably between ages forty-five and fifty. Also, when you are pregnant, you do not have a period. And many women who nurse their new babies (feed them milk from their breasts) do not start having periods again until they stop nursing their babies.

Q "Can I stay home from school?"

A No. Remember, this is not an illness, it is normal life. You can keep your typical schedule and do almost any activity. You may feel a little out of sorts the first day or two. That's natural. Those wonderful hormones are working hard, and you'll feel the effects. Try not to snap at your friends and family. There may be some pain in your abdomen, but it shouldn't last long. You may hear this pain called "the cramps." Some girls use them as an excuse to do nothing. Most of you will feel better if you are busy and don't focus on these pains. Many of you will not even have the cramps during your period. If you have severe pain, talk with your mother and a doctor.

Girls, I think you can understand everything I've said about menstruation. You also need to know that it's an incredibly complex process thought up by our Master Designer, by God.

And fellas, you need to be reminded of this, too. Understanding sexuality means understanding what it means to be male *and* female. So, if you skimmed over these last few paragraphs, go back and really read them. And girls, for the same reason, you keep on reading.

Boys, let's talk a bit about wet dreams. Sounds interesting doesn't, it? And no, we're *not* talking about falling asleep in the shower or camping in a rainstorm! We *are* talking about a physical signal that your body is changing from a boy's to a man's body.

Boys, let me anticipate your questions about all this, and give you some answers, too.

Q **"Start with the basics here, and tell me how this happens."**

A A good, no-nonsense approach. Do you remember the list of body changes you could expect? Your testicles and your penis will grow bigger. These changes prepare your sexual organs for the next step in their growth—making sperm cells. Your body makes a milky-like fluid which makes it easier to pass the sperm cells.

When the sperm mix with the fluid, it is called semen.

You know that urine flows out of your penis, too. But when the semen flows out, the urine is blocked from the penis. The passing of semen is called ejaculation.

When you were younger, you probably noticed your penis became erect every now and then. It would become hard and stand out from your body and soon become limp and soft again. As you grow, having an erection also means an ejaculation sometimes occurs. The first time this happens, you will most likely be asleep. When you wake up, you'll notice the semen on your pajamas. This will be your first wet dream. You will have these during your teenage years.

You'll be surprised, and the wet spots will be a bit sticky. But the semen is harmless. Simply wipe it off. You may want to change your pajamas. There is no need to be embarrassed, guys. Your parents know this is normal for a growing, changing boy.

Q **"I want to be ready for this. When will it happen?"**

A An important detail. Some of you will have your first wet dream around age twelve. Others may have your first around age fifteen or anytime in between.

Q **"Why does this happen? And why in my sleep?"**

A Remember, I mentioned that your body cannot store the sperm cells it produces; they must be passed out of your body. As you change, there will be a sort of tension that builds inside of you before the sperm are released. Because you're changing, this tension sometimes prompts a pleasurable dream during your sleep (most often about a girl). Your body's response, acting without your thinking about it, will make your penis erect and an ejaculation of semen will occur. The tension is released, and your penis becomes soft and limp again. It is a very natural way your body handles its sexual tension.

Q **"Ok, so it's normal. Aren't there any other normal ways to handle this?"**

A Very good question, and the answer is *yes*. Read carefully, though.

Intercourse, when a man's erect penis is inside a woman's vagina, is a chance for a natural release. Semen is then ejaculated into the woman's uterus. This is an act God intended only for husbands and wives (Gen. 2:24). The Bible is clear on that.

We'd better talk about one other release—masturbation. This occurs when you rub your hand up and down your penis. Your penis becomes erect, and you may bring on an ejaculation of semen, too.

Boys, you have touched your penis or stroked or rubbed it since you were an infant. This is a normal kind of self-discovery. You were curious about your body. To rub your penis felt good.

The greatest pleasure from God's gift of sex is giving pleasure to another person, showing deep love for another person. It is *not* giving pleasure to yourself. Masturbation only focuses on you. If you masturbate, you encourage yourself to be selfish and misuse God's gift to you.

Girls (you have been reading all along, haven't you?), you also masturbate, by rubbing your clitoris, a small spot above your urethra. It brings the same kind of pleasant physical feelings that boys have rubbing their penises. And just like boys, you run the risk of selfishness if you choose this behavior. Reread the last paragraph.

Boys and girls, realize that masturbation now and in the next few years is not the same as a curious child exploring his body. Masturbation is a selfish act. Be sure and talk this over with parents or adult friends. They can reassure you. The better you understand your sexuality, the less need you will have to do it.

So, let's keep reading!

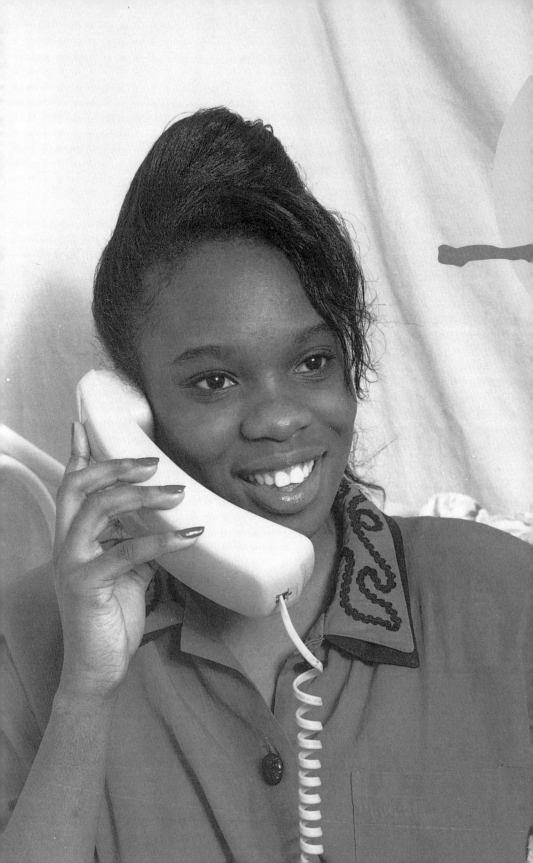

My Feelings— Where They Come From

I've come to a decision. This is one of the best times of your life. Many things are going your way. You're not a *little* kid anymore, you're a *big* kid! You probably have two or three best friends you can count on. Your church offers you more to do and learn. This is likely a fairly peaceful time with your parents, too.

Why would anyone want to give all this up?

LET'S...

◆ About Jesus, Luke wrote:

> "Jesus grew in wisdom and stature, and in favor with God and men" (Luke 2:52, NIV).

Jesus once was your age. I know you *know* that, but let it really sink in. Jesus didn't stay a baby in the manger. Jesus grew each year just as all children grow... just as *you* grow.

◆ The Bible also teaches us that Jesus understands human life. Jesus understands us. Jesus sympathizes with our weaknesses; He was "tempted in every way, just as we are—yet without sin" (Heb. 4:15, NIV). Since Jesus was once your age, He understands about being your age. That's important news. But do you know what the next most important news is? He understands what it's like to be a year older, two years older, three years older. You don't have to be afraid to change; Jesus can help you through all these changes.

◆ There's another important Bible verse to think on. The verse is from a letter the prophet Jeremiah sent to the people in exile in Babylon.

In the letter the prophet gives God's message to the people. The verse is a promise of hope that speaks to us today.

God's plans for you are good plans, the best plans. If you stay your age today, you'll never know the good that God has planned for you. His plan is a future filled with hope.

"Does that mean my life always will be filled with good things? Are change and growing up always happy and fun?" you may ask. My, you ask good questions! I'd like to promise you that, but I know better. And you know better, too, don't you? Life isn't always fair. You've lived long enough to see that's true.

Boys and girls, there's one thing better than fair, and it is this: **knowing my life is in God's care and that my life pleases Him**.

Life is not always fair, but *God* is. *Every change* may not *seem* good, but God can help you *find something good* in the change.

We've already talked about some of the changes headed your way. Just remember: you and change will get along just fine. Jesus lived through the changes, too. You can deal with changes, such as a squeaky voice, clumsy feet, strange inner feelings, and all. And God is with you.

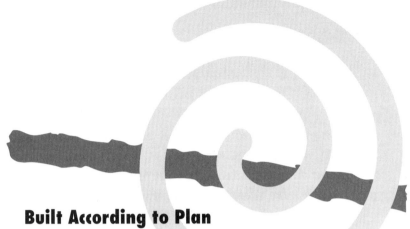

Built According to Plan

Up until now, there haven't been very many physical differences between you and your friends, boys or girls. Have you noticed? Younger boys and girls have about the same body shape. Inside, they have the same major organs, like the heart, liver, lungs, and brain.

Everyone has sexual organs, too. But they *are* different for boys and girls.

You were born with these sexual organs. But they do not begin to function until **puberty** begins. Remember the pop-up timer? And those hormones from the pituitary gland? That's the beginning of changes in your body. Your sexual organs then begin to make other hormones that prompt the changes in those organs and in your feelings about being male and female. Welcome to puberty!

You're going to hear (if you haven't already) some kids your age make jokes about sex, the sexual organs, and the sexual relationship between men and women. It's OK to talk about and ask questions about those things. But the kids telling the jokes will be making fun of these good things. They may use crude language and slang words. Many times, it is because they do not know the correct words or understand how their bodies function or why they feel these new feelings inside them.

These kinds of jokes may seem harmless. But don't forget this. Your body is part of God's creation. They way it functions is His design. Disrespect for what God created is disrespect for God. Don't let your friends trick you into going along with such talk.

Getting Back to Those Feelings...

We started by talking about change—and how we feel about it. Remember Matthew and Kristin and their friends? We've seen how they are changing. Let's see how they're *feeling* about those changes.

The bodies of Zac and Rachel have started changing before their friends' bodies have begun to change. Sometimes they think they are better than others their same ages. Sometimes (though they won't admit it), they are very self-conscious about their growing bodies. They don't look like their friends, and they feel like they stick out in the crowd—like a sore thumb. Their snooty behavior at times is probably a way to cover up how uncomfortable and different they feel.

Zac and Rachel need to remember that changing earlier does *not* make them better. So do their friends. So do you, especially if you have one of those bodies in a hurry to start changing.

Phil and Casy are the group's grouches, fighting with parents and friends. Their hormones are sending lots of chemical messages throughout their bodies. Sometimes they feel confused. Sometimes they feel real physical pain. They seem to snap at everyone then.

Phil and Casy need to remember that talking about these confusing changes, especially with parents or other caring adults, helps everyone. Believe it or not, adults remember how they felt at your age and during puberty. Most of them will tell you they have no desire to live through it again. They remember, and they understand.

Kristin and her best friends often feel embarrassed about being taller than others their age, especially being taller than the boys. They need to remember that most girls have growth spurts before boys do, and everyone grows at different times and at different rates. And, for the next few years, you girls will probably be interested in boyfriends *before* you boys are interested in girlfriends. Kristin may go through a year or two of having a crush on boys older than she is. Then, when the boys her age are ready to like her and her friends, they might feel frustrated because the girls aren't interested in them.

Kristin and her friends, and you too, will probably be happier getting to know lots of boys and enjoying being friends with them. As a preadolescent you have enough to do just figuring out what your body is doing. That's why its best not to be limited to *one* boyfriend or *one* girlfriend.

Michael and Jessica are good examples of the problems with growth spurts, too. She feels unhappy and embarrassed when she's clumsy. He is tired so often he hardly feels anything except hungry.

Michael and Jessica need to remember that these awkward times come and go and don't last long. And they happen as everybody grows.

Then there's Jonathan, the group's Romeo. He's feeling the effects of hormones from his pituitary gland and testicles. These hormones stir a new kind of excited feeling inside, especially when Jonathan is near Jessica or thinking about any girl.

This is another important part of changing into men and women. New feelings you've never had before come with these changes. The feelings are normal and, like your body's growing, they are automatic. Jonathan needs to remember that your attitudes and actions about your changing body, your sexuality, and others' sexuality, are entirely up to you. Here's where the real challenge is. And I think you're ready to meet the challenge. Read on!

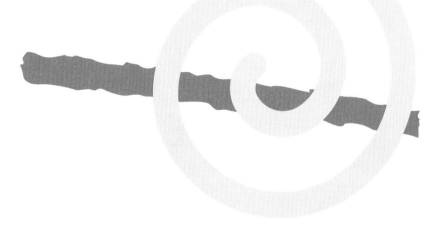

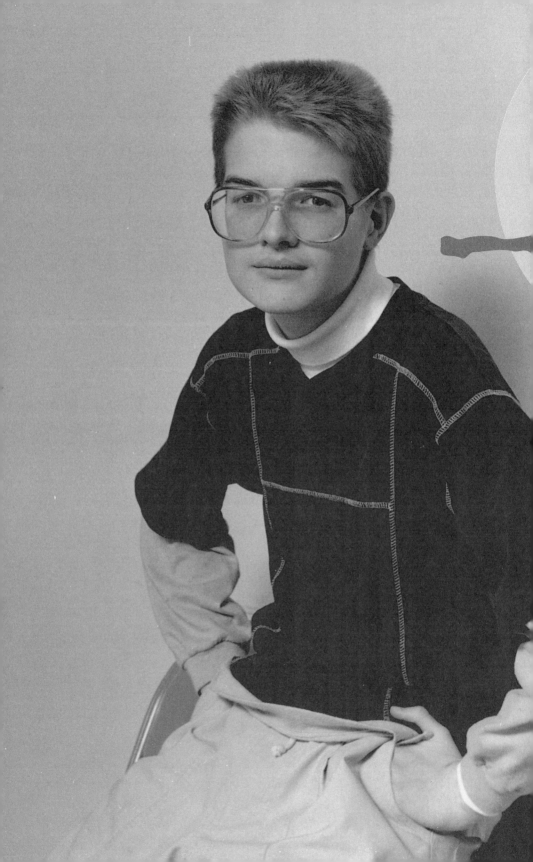

My Attitudes—
My Business!

"You need an attitude adjustment." Has your parent or teacher ever said this to you?

We've covered *a lot of information* about you, your body, and your sexuality. Knowing all of it is important. How you think and act because of it is even *more* important.

"Even a child is known by his actions, by whether his conduct is pure and right" (Prov. 20:11, NIV).

In each chapter, I've asked you to "think on these things" from the Bible. Anything we learn from the Bible changes our thoughts and our actions. If it doesn't, we *really haven't learned it.*

Your attitudes about sex are your inner thoughts and ideas about sex. Attitudes are based on the information you allow into your mind. Let's take a moment to check out your **sources of information** about sex. Let's see how they might affect your attitudes.

◆ Your friends

They are more important to you than ever before. And, as we've already talked about, becoming curious about sex is normal for kids your age. Naturally, your friends may talk about it a lot. Funny thing, though, these conversations usually are very secretive. Why do your friends want to whisper and giggle about sex and pretend sex is a secret?

Well, it's fun to talk about stuff that you keep

secret from parents or other adults. It makes you closer to your friends. And your friends may be showing off a little by whispering some new "fact" that no one else knows about sex.

Just don't believe everything you hear. Sometimes your friends are telling dirty jokes or using bad language. They've heard it from someone else, probably older, and want to shock you with it. They're not concerned whether it's true or false.

Some of your friends have not been carefully learning about their sexuality like you have with this book. *Some* of their parents aren't discussing sex with them like yours may be. And *some* have never heard what God says about sex. So, *some* of their information will not be accurate or biblical. Their attitudes may be that sex is a dirty secret that you tell in crude words. *They* need an attitude adjustment. If you depend on friends for your sexual information, you could be misled.

◆ Television, movies, magazines, newspapers—the media

The folks producing all these things have learned that people watch more, listen more, want more, buy more when sex is included. You see and hear many sexual messages in the media. Be very careful about what you watch and hear and what you believe. You see, your friends may tell you wrong information because they don't know yet what is right. But most folks sending media messages are adults. When sex is part of their message, they sometimes make it appear selfish, ugly, or violent *on purpose*. They want you to believe that anyone can act or talk "sexy" anytime they want. And they want you to believe that people who use certain soaps, drive certain cars, or wear certain clothes are sexy people that everyone else will want to be with and to be like.

If you accept their messages, you will easily accept their version of sex, too. Remember, the media isn't trying to teach you a healthy view of sexuality. They're trying to sell you records, movies, and advertisers' products. Ask yourself: Does this agree with the Bible's words on sex? Do I care if my parents see or hear this? Would I honor God if I talked or acted the same way?

◆ Sex education

Most schools include discussions about sex. Schools approach this subject in different ways. They may teach about body changes and growth, the names and work of the sex organs, and how babies grow and are born. They also may teach about sexually transmitted diseases (called STDs), AIDS, and sexual crimes.

Your parents are interested in what your school teaches you about sex. They usually won't know when you are in sex education classes or what you're taught. Plan to tell them about these studies just like you tell them about math tests, science fair projects, games during P.E., and other classes. You and your family will want to test the ideas taught in your school's sex education classes by God's Word. Trusted adults can help you sort through all the information you receive.

I feel like I'm telling you: "Don't trust just anyone's information on sex!" Does it seem that way to you, too? What I mean to say is this. There are many mixed-up people with mixed-up sexual messages. Some of these people are nice people but do not have correct information. The values of some people will be different from the values you hold. You know some of these people, but others are strangers. Get correct information and think carefully and prayerfully about sex and sexuality. If you do not, you may need a sexual attitude adjustment.

GET OFF TO A GOOD START ON YOUR ATTITUDES...

THINK ON THESE THINGS

▼ Jesus said:

"The good man brings good things out of the good stored up in him, and the evil man brings evil things out of the evil stored up in him" (Matt. 12:35, NIV).

That verse reminds me of a computer phrase: **garbage in, garbage out**! You will have a good, healthy attitude about sex if you store good, healthy information inside you and use the information properly.

▼ God creates all people, but He uses men and women to do this. When a man's penis is erect, he can fit it into a woman's vagina. The semen he ejaculates inside her sends millions of sperm cells into her uterus. If one sperm joins one of the woman's egg cells in her fallopian tubes, it will settle in the lining of the uterus. The sperm cell and the egg cell form one cell. From that cell a baby will grow. In about nine months the baby will be born. Remember, God said to Adam and Eve:

"Be fruitful and increase in number;
fill the earth" (Gen. 1:28, NIV).

"Have children," God was saying to them, "as part of My purpose for your lives."

▼ God's plan is for children to be born to a husband and wife who love each other. The story of Samuel's birth is a beautiful example of this. Samuel's parents prayed many years for a child. The Bible says Elkanah loved Hannah (1 Sam. 1:5) and comforted her when it seemed they never would have a child (1 Sam. 1:8). Hannah prayed for a child. Hannah gave birth to a son. She named him Samuel, saying, "Because I asked the Lord for him." This loving couple knew God had given them this son. Their act of sexual intercourse was only one part of the love and care they expressed for each other. Samuel's parents loved God and loved each other before he was born.

The birth of each child shows God's love for that child. And the birth of each child shows the love of a husband and wife for each other. This kind of love is made known in many ways. Sex is only one of the many ways.

▼ God also wants you and every person born to be born again. Jesus once helped a man understand being born again in John 3:3-8,16-18. Jesus died in our place for our sins. To be born again you must turn from sin as a way of life and trust Jesus as your Lord and Savior. As a Christian, you are God's creation—again.

SO...

THINK ON THESE THINGS

When a friend tells a dirty joke, YOU THINK ON *THESE* THINGS.

When television and movies show unmarried people having sex for selfish reasons, YOU THINK ON *THESE* THINGS.

When your sex education class at school leaves out the importance of marriage for sexual expression, YOU THINK ON *THESE* THINGS.

When you hear about victims of terrible sexual crimes or abuse, YOU THINK ON *THESE* THINGS.

After all, no one else will watch out for your attitudes. Your attitudes are your business.

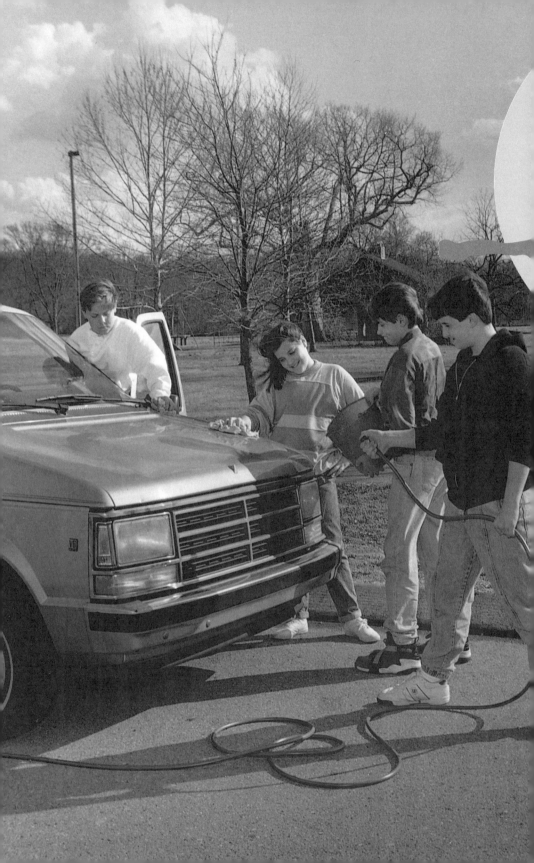

My Actions—In Control and On Course

I've tried to be very honest with you in these last four chapters. I feel like you're at such an important age, this in-between age. And you need answers to many questions. I've tried to share with you how special you are to God, and how wonderful it is to think about sexuality the way He does.

Well, I've got to be honest with you in this last chapter, too. And the truth is—

you live in a world where everything is not as God intended. Check out the headlines in any newspaper, listen to the lead story on the evening news, talk to your school's guidance counselor, visit your city's courtrooms, even take a look around your neighborhood. People have so many ways to hurt and abuse other people that it boggles your mind. And because so many people, including grown people, think about sex as a dirty secret or as a selfish way to get what they want, many rotten things that happen involve sex.

Kids, it is as important as *life and death* that you decide right now, as a ten- or eleven-year-old or twelve-or-thirteen-year-old, to keep your life **in control** and **on course**. If you make that commitment about your sexuality, you will find your life stays in control and on course in every other area as well.

The Facts

Here are some facts about some things that happen in your world:

◆ More than one million teenage girls get pregnant every year. This means that more than one million teenage boys are involved, too.

◆ Almost half of the teenagers who go to church have sexual intercourse.

◆ Some children your age are forced or tricked into a sexual relationship with an adult. Sometimes an adult might touch a child's sexual parts or make the child touch the adult's sexual parts. An adult might even have sexual intercourse with a child. These acts are called **sexual abuse.** Here is the saddest part; the adult who does these things to a child is usually the child's parent or another family member or relative. Child abuse is against the law. It is wrong for an adult to force this behavior on a child. If this happens to you, tell someone.

◆ Some people teach that marriage is old-fashioned. Worse, some believe marriage is only a religious belief that cannot be taught in schools or protected by our country's laws.

◆ Some teenagers in high school and in college make fun of others who admit they are virgins. (A virgin is a boy or girl who waits until marriage to have sexual intercourse.) It is God's plan for boys and girls to remain a virgin until marriage.

This kind of world is sad and it's scary to live in.

Once More Through the Garden...

Think again about God's creation of Adam and Eve. We've learned many truths from these early verses in the Bible:

- that God made us
- that our sexuality is a part of God's plan
- that our sexuality is His way to bring children into families
- that marriage is the only place where sexual intercourse belongs

Let's add one more truth.

● God loves people so much He gave them freedom to choose. Freedom to choose is a great gift. Here's what the Bible says:

> "The Lord God took the man and put him in the Garden of Eden to work it and take care of it. And the Lord God commanded the man, 'You are free to eat from any tree in the garden, but you must not eat from the tree of the knowledge of good and evil, for when you eat of it you will surely die' " (Gen. 2:15-17, NIV).

Some days, you may wish you did not have to choose. I mean, if I didn't have to choose, I would not be responsible for my actions. I wouldn't be tempted to do wrong actions because I could not choose. At times you may wish God had made people to do only right.

People were created in "the image of God." Being made in the image of God means, among other things, that people can choose and are responsible for their choices. People are not robots. Animals act by instinct or because of training. People can reason and make choices.

God loves us, but we can choose not to love Him. He wants us to know Him, but we can choose to ignore Him. God wants us to make wise and right choices, but we can choose to go our own way. God will not force us to do right.

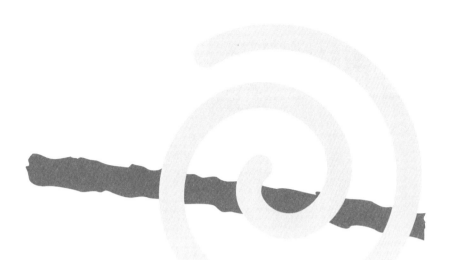

Some of our choices lead us to sin. Sin is like shooting at a target and missing it. We sin when we miss God's plan for us by doing things our own way.

Sin has a price tag on it. The Bible is clear about this:

"Do not be deceived: God cannot be mocked. A man reaps what he sows" (Gal. 6:7, NIV).

It's like this. A farmer who plants wheat expects wheat to grow. He expects to harvest wheat.

If you plant sinful thoughts and attitudes in your life, you can expect sinful behavior to grow from them. And you will pay sin's terrible price—guaranteed.

So, read on carefully.

CHOOSE CAREFULLY TO STAY IN CONTROL...

▼ An important goal should be to grow as Christ wants you to grow. As you try to live as Jesus wants you to live your life will produce *this* "fruit":

> "love, joy, peace, patience, kindness, goodness, faithfulness, gentleness, and self-control" (Gal. 5:22-23, NIV).

It sounds impossible, but you gain control of your life when you give control to God. There's no other way to be like Him.

And don't miss this: It is easier to control your actions when you control your words. Paul wrote these words to some first-century Christians:

> "Nor should there be obscenity, foolish talk or coarse joking, which are out of place" (Eph. 5:4, NIV).

If you or your friends are telling dirty jokes about sex, if you're using slang words for parts of your body or someone else's body, *that's out of place!*

These are the words King David wrote about the importance of what we say:

> "May the words of my mouth and the meditation of my heart be pleasing in your sight, O Lord, my Rock and my Redeemer" (Ps. 19:4, NIV).

Do you know what that says to me? If I don't *talk about* sinful stuff, I'm less likely to *do* sinful stuff. Why? Because my mind is thinking on other things.

Is this starting to sink in? I hope so. An old proverb says, "Sticks and stones may break my bones, but words will never hurt me." Boys and girls, that's just not so. Your words can hurt you or other people—deep, wounding hurts. It matters how you talk about sex for the same reasons.

▼ One more encouragement to control your actions. You may hear someone say, "Sex is only an instinct. You're born with it. So whatever you feel like doing—*do it!*" This is the old "let nature take its course" argument, and it's baloney.

You *are* a sexual person, male or female. Your body is changing (or will begin to change soon). You are or soon will be more aware of *being* male or female. With the changes come new, natural instincts—boys interested in girls, girls interested in boys.

Now, think a minute. Guys, you see a girl at

the mall who stirs your interest. Your instinct is to grab her and kiss her immediately. What do you tell the mall's security officer who runs over? "She's so great to look at, I just followed my natural instincts and expressed my sexual interest in her."

He'll say, "Nice try, kid, but no cigar."

You aren't a slave to the instincts of your body. Animals are, but you aren't.

The instinct to be sexually close to a person does not give you the right to act. This is a signal that your body is preparing for the time when you will love one person. You have much to learn about the strong commitment necessary for loving one person. You're still a long way from marriage.

So, any action which misuses your sexuality or another's before marriage is wrong. Paul told the Christians at Corinth:

> "The body is not meant for sexual immorality, but for the Lord, and the Lord for the body" (1 Cor. 6:13b, NIV).

Remember how much God loves you and how perfect is His creation of you. When you use your body, mind, and feelings the way God created you to use them, you show the best kind of love for Him, for yourself, and for others.

Paul went on to say:

"Avoid sexual looseness like the plague! Every other sin that a man commits is done outside his own body, but this is an offense against his own body. Have you forgotten . . . that you are not the owner of your own body? You have been bought, and at a price! Therefore bring glory to God in your body" (1 Cor. 6:18-20, Phillips).

Let's sum up then. We keep our actions in control by:
● giving control of our lives to God
● controlling what we say
● refusing to sin against our own bodies

Out of Control...

The city where I live is in a hilly area. The streets have many unusual twists and turns. Finding new places in town is sometimes hard to do. Many times, I've found myself staring at a street sign that says **DEAD END** or **NO OUTLET**. I know if I turn down that street, I'll be going nowhere.

Boys and girls, if you are sexually out of control, you'll be sending your life down a dead-end road. If you have sexual intercourse before you're married, you may be stuck in one of these dead ends:

Pregnancy

Girls as young as eight have become pregnant. In fact, girls, you can become pregnant six months before your first period even starts. Pregnancy at your age is a tragedy. Your body isn't strong enough or big enough to carry a baby in it. The baby will probably be very small and sick even if you can carry it for nine months. Babies need to come home to a loving mother and father who are ready to care for a baby. Boys and girls your age cannot provide these.

Boys, pregnancy is not just a girl's problem. No girl ever became pregnant without a boy supplying the sperm that fertilized an egg inside her. If you are the father of the child, you are just as responsible for pregnancy as the girl.

Homosexuality

People who prefer sexual activity with partners of the same sex are known as homosexuals. Men who prefer men are called gays. Women who prefer women are known as lesbians.

Homosexuality is not new. It was practiced in the pagan world, especially in Rome, but the Jewish religion held up God's will for male and female to mate. The Bible contains laws condemning sexual misuses, including homosexuality. (See Lev. 18—21.)

In Romans 1:26-32 and 1 Corinthians 6:9, Paul condemned homosexuality as violating God's plan for man and woman to complete one another sexually.

At this in-between time in the lives of preadolescents, bodies are developing sexually. Some preadolescents may be confused about their sexual feelings. It is not unusual for boys and girls of this age to prefer friends of the same sex. That does not mean those boys and girls are homosexuals.

STD's

STD stands for sexually transmitted diseases. These are diseases spread through sexual contact. Some names you may hear are gonorrhea, herpes, or chlamydia. Some are easy to treat; some have no cure. Some make sores you can see; some don't. Some are fatal. The *only* sure way to avoid STD's is to avoid sexual contact.

This means more than just saying NO to sexual intercourse. Some STD's are spread when you touch any part of your body to the infection on someone else's body. You could become sick by touching an infected person's clothing or hands, especially if those have been in contact with their infection. Some STD's appear in the mouth, and they are spread by kissing.

Finally, remember this. Anyone who infects you with an STD has been sexually active with one or more other persons. They probably are not interested in the special, splendid, God-created you. They are more interested in using you for their sexual purposes. That's not the kind of person you want to develop a friendship with anyway.

AIDS

AIDS stands for acquired immune deficiency syndrome. You've heard a lot about AIDS. AIDS is something you should fear. Why?

AIDS is sneaky. You may not know you have AIDS until ten years after you are infected. If you were sexually active during those ten years, you could infect every sexual partner you have. So could the person who infected you. What a tragedy.

AIDS is deadly. On this day as I write, there is no cure for AIDS. *Every AIDS patient dies.* Even if a cure is found, the threat will not be gone for a long time. Remember, you can have the disease years before it begins to make you sick. Once AIDS destroys your immune system (that's your body's ability to fight disease and infection), it is gone forever. If you get AIDS, your body simply cannot fight off disease and infections.

I started this chapter by saying your actions regarding sex could mean life or death. Now you know why.

USE YOUR CHOICES TO STAY ON COURSE...

▼ The easiest way to stay on course is to follow directions. Even in unfamiliar places, you can get where you want to go by following the road signs or by reading a map.

You have a perfect set of directions to keep your life on course. It is the Bible:

"How can a young man keep his way pure? By living according to your word. I seek you with my whole heart; do not let me stray from your commands" (Ps. 119:9-10, NIV).

"Turn my eyes away from worthless things; preserve my life according to your word. Your hands made me and formed me; give me understanding to learn your commands. Your word, O Lord, is eternal; ...you established the earth, and it endures. Your laws endure to this day." (Ps. 119:37, 73, 89*a*, 90*b*-91,

Jesus faced Satan's toughest temptations by remembering Scripture. Read about it in Matthew 4.

When many followers deserted Jesus, He asked His twelve disciples if they would desert Him. Peter said to Him,

> "Lord, to whom shall we go? You have the words of eternal life" (John 6:68, NIV).

Choose life by knowing and practicing God's Word. The teachings of the Bible can keep you *on course*.

▼ Stay on course by planning ahead. Solomon said:

> "Those who plan what is good find love and faithfulness" (Prov. 14:22, NIV).

You need to decide *today* to have a marriage of love and faithfulness. If you decide those things now, then you've also decided:

—to respect your body and to care for it

—to respect others and speak only good words about them

—to respect God's plan for your sexuality and wait for marriage before you have sexual intercourse

▼ You're not too young to choose God's plan for your life. In fact, I would encourage you with the same words that Paul used to encourage his young friend, Timothy:

"Don't let anyone look down on you because you are young, but set an example for the believers in speech, in life, in love, in faith and in purity" (1 Tim. 4:12, NIV).

Purity refers specifically to being sexually pure, to avoiding all sexual sins. Your decision to stay pure not only benefits you, it can be an example for others to follow. Even kids older than you. Even adults.

Getting Off Course Can Happen If...

... you're in the wrong place. A friend's party without his parents at home is the wrong place. R-rated and X-rated movie theaters are the wrong place.

... you've got the wrong stuff. Drugs and alcohol are the wrong stuff—many who become sexually active say they are drunk or high when they are having sexual intercourse. Pornographic magazines are the wrong stuff. Women are used rather than respected. Women are used to excite men's interest in sex. Often pictures show women and children being beaten or abused through some type of sexual activity. These magazines are the worst kind of trash. Don't look at them. When your friends get copies, walk away. One look is too many.

.... you're with the wrong people. I've told you that your friends can be a problem, with their latest dirty joke, with their misinformation. Be considerate of all people, but be careful about forming your friendships. Kids you think are your friends may ask you to try sexual things on your body or on their body. That's not the request of a real friend.

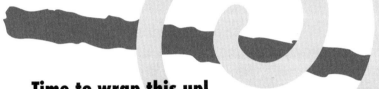

Time to wrap this up!

I have mixed feelings as our talk comes to an end. On the one hand, I feel like we have covered it all. There's nothing more to say. But on the other hand, I know there is so much more that you need to know, just not right now. As you leave your tweenage years and head toward your teenage years, much of what we have talked about will really start to make sense.

Keep learning about God's wonderful gift to you of sexuality. Stay in places and with people who will support your decision to honor God with your sexuality.

I have one final suggestion for you, especially to keep your actions in control and on course. Begin now to pray for the husband or wife God may someday bring into your life. Ask Him now to protect that person and keep that person pure. Ask Him to protect you and keep you pure.

The apostle Paul has helped us with many important truths about sexuality. I think I'll give him the final word on the subject:

"It is God's will that you should be sanctified: that you should avoid sexual immorality; that each of you should learn to control his own body in a way that is holy and honorable, not in passionate lust like the heathen, who do not know God; and that in this matter no one should wrong his brother or take advantage of him. The Lord will punish men for all such sins, as we have already told you and warned you. For God did not call us to be impure, but to live a holy life. Therefore, he who rejects this instruction does not reject man but God, who gives you his Holy Spirit" (1 Thess. 4:3-8, NIV).

My Journal— Ideas and Questions

Use the following pages as a kind of journal to record new ideas you discovered when reading each chapter. Also, write down any questions that you still need answered. But, don't just write them down, talk with your parent or a trusted adult friend and get answers to your questions.

Preadolescent— and Proud of It

New ideas I discovered...

_____

_____

_____

_____

_____

Questions I still need answered...

_____

_____

_____

_____

_____

_____

_____

My Body— What It Means to Be Me

New ideas I discovered...

_____

_____

_____

_____

_____

Questions I still need answered...

_____

_____

_____

_____

_____

_____

My Growing—
Understanding
God's Timing

New ideas I discovered...

_____

_____

_____

_____

_____

Questions I still need answered...

_____

_____

_____

_____

_____

_____

My Feelings— Where They Come From

New ideas I discovered...

_____

_____

_____

_____

_____

Questions I still need answered...

_____

_____

_____

_____

_____

_____

My Attitudes— My Business!

New ideas I discovered...

_____

_____

_____

_____

_____

Questions I still need answered...

_____

_____

_____

_____

_____

_____

_____

My Actions—
In Control and
On Course

New ideas I discovered...

_____

_____

_____

_____

_____

Questions I still need answered...

_____

_____

_____

_____

_____

_____